Health worker roles in providing
safe abortion care and post-abortion contraception

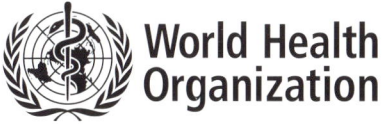

Acknowledgements

The guideline was developed by the Department of Reproductive Health and Research, World Health Organization.

We acknowledge the many staff and consultants to the Department who contributed towards this effort. We thank the staff of the Norwegian Knowledge Centre for the Health Services, Oslo, Norway, for their work in evidence synthesis and assessment, and the Norwegian Agency for Development Cooperation for supporting the staff's time to work on this project.

We are also deeply grateful to the members of the Guideline Development Group and the external peer reviewers.

A complete list of contributors and their specific roles can be found in Annex A: Contributors to the guideline.

Editing, design and layout by Green Ink (greenink.co.uk)

Cover design by J. Petitpierre

WHO Library Cataloguing-in-Publication Data

Health worker roles in providing safe abortion care and post abortion contraception.

Contents: 3 web supplements: Evidence-to-Decision (EtD) Frameworks 2015 – Annex Nos.1-26: Evidence base for benefits and harms – Annexes 27-40: acceptability and feasibility

1.Abortion, Induced. 2.Contraception. 3.Health Personnel. 4.Guideline. I.World Health Organization.

ISBN 978 92 4 154926 4   (NLM classification: WQ 440)

© World Health Organization 2015

All rights reserved. Publications of the World Health Organization are available on the WHO website (www.who.int) or can be purchased from WHO Press, World Health Organization, 20 Avenue Appia, 1211 Geneva 27, Switzerland (tel.: +41 22 791 3264; fax: +41 22 791 4857; e-mail: bookorders@who.int).

Requests for permission to reproduce or translate WHO publications –whether for sale or for non-commercial distribution– should be addressed to WHO Press through the WHO website (www.who.int/about/licensing/copyright_form/en/index.html).

The designations employed and the presentation of the material in this publication do not imply the expression of any opinion whatsoever on the part of the World Health Organization concerning the legal status of any country, territory, city or area or of its authorities, or concerning the delimitation of its frontiers or boundaries. Dotted and dashed lines on maps represent approximate border lines for which there may not yet be full agreement.

The mention of specific companies or of certain manufacturers' products does not imply that they are endorsed or recommended by the World Health Organization in preference to others of a similar nature that are not mentioned. Errors and omissions excepted, the names of proprietary products are distinguished by initial capital letters.

All reasonable precautions have been taken by the World Health Organization to verify the information contained in this publication. However, the published material is being distributed without warranty of any kind, either expressed or implied. The responsibility for the interpretation and use of the material lies with the reader. In no event shall the World Health Organization be liable for damages arising from its use.

Printed in Spain.

Contents

Acronyms and abbreviations	**v**
Executive summary	**1**
Rationale for this guideline	3
Process of guideline development	4
Overview of recommendations	4
Research needs	11
Update and review	11
Tasks and health workers considered in the guideline	**12**
Background	**15**
Shortage of health-care professionals	17
Effective, safe and simple interventions exist for safe abortion and post-abortion care	17
Other relevant global guidelines	19
Objectives of this guideline	19
How the guideline was developed	**21**
Contributors and their roles	23
Scoping and formulation of the guideline questions	24
Evidence retrieval and synthesis	24
Assessment of confidence in the evidence	26
Moving from evidence to recommendations	26
Recommendations	**29**
General considerations	31
Recommendation categories	32
Management of abortion and post-abortion care for pregnancies in the first trimester	33
Management of abortion and post-abortion care for pregnancies beyond 12 weeks	45
Management of non-life-threatening complications	53
Information about safe abortion and contraception	55
Pre- and post-abortion counselling	56
Provision of post-abortion contraception	57

Research needs and implementation considerations — 65
Research needs — 67
General implementation considerations — 67

Guideline dissemination, adaptation, monitoring and review — 69
Dissemination and adaptation of the guideline — 71
Monitoring guideline use — 71
Review and update of the guideline — 71

References — 73

Annex A: Contributors to the guideline — 77

Supplementary material

The following supplementary material is available as web-based annexes at www.who.int/reproductivehealth/publications/unsafe_abortion/abortion-task-shifting/en/.

Web Supplement 1:
Evidence to Decision (EtD) frameworks

- This supplement provides a summary of the evidence and information that informed the recommendations and the process by which the recommendation decisions were made.

Web Supplement 2:
Annexes 1–26: Evidence base for benefits and harms

- This supplement provides a summary of all systematic reviews, search strategies, Summary of Findings tables and GRADE tables, as well as the detailed PICOs.

Web Supplement 3:
Annexes 27–40: Evidence base for acceptability and feasibility

- This supplement provides a summary of all qualitative systematic reviews, search strategies, Summary of Findings tables and CERQual assessments.

Acronyms and abbreviations

AN	auxiliary nurse
ANM	auxiliary nurse midwife
CERQual	Confidence in the Evidence from Reviews of Qualitative Research
CINAHL	Cumulative Index to Nursing and Allied Health Literature
DECIDE	Developing and Evaluating Communication Strategies to Support Informed Decisions and Practice Based on Evidence
D&E	dilatation and evacuation
DOI	declaration of interest
Embase	Excerpta Medica database
EmOC	emergency obstetric care
EtD	Evidence to Decision
EVA	electric vacuum aspiration
FIGO	Fédération Internationale de Gynécologie et d'Obstétrique (International Federation of Gynecology and Obstetrics)
GDG	Guideline Development Group
GRADE	Grading of Recommendations Assessment, Development and Evaluation
IM	intramuscular
IUD	intrauterine device
IV	intravenous
LILACS	Literatura Latinoamericana y del Caribe en Ciencias de la Salud
MA	medical abortion
MNH	maternal and newborn health
MVA	manual vacuum aspiration
NGO	nongovernmental organization
PAHO	Pan American Health Organization
PICO	population, intervention, comparator, outcome
RHL	WHO Reproductive Health Library
UNFPA	United Nations Population Fund
USA	United States of America
WHO	World Health Organization

Executive summary

Tasks and health workers

Executive summary

Moving beyond specialist doctors to involve a wider range of health workers is an increasingly important public health strategy. Planned and regulated task shifting and task sharing can ensure a rational optimization of the available health workforce, address health system shortages of specialized health-care professionals, improve equity in access to health care and increase the acceptability of health services for those receiving them.

Rationale for this guideline

Although safe, simple and effective evidence-based interventions exist, nearly 22 million unsafe abortions take place every year; these continue to contribute significantly to the global burden of maternal mortality and morbidity.

Among the many barriers that limit access to safe abortion care, the lack of trained providers is one of the most critical. It is estimated that the global deficit of skilled health-care professionals will reach 12.9 million by 2035. Such shortages are especially critical in regions of the world that also have a high burden of unsafe abortion and related mortality. Additionally, most countries, including many high-income ones, have subnational disparities in the availability of a skilled health workforce, with shortages being particularly high in rural areas or within the public sector.

Policy and regulatory barriers, stigma or the unwillingness of some health-care professionals to provide care may further limit the availability of safe abortion and post-abortion care providers in many contexts. This leaves particular subpopulations of women – for example, rural, less educated, poor, adolescent or unmarried women – at risk of unsafe abortion.

Although in many contexts abortion-related care provision is limited to specialist doctors, many of the evidence-based interventions for safe abortion and post-abortion care, particularly those in early pregnancy, can be provided on an outpatient basis at the primary care level. The emergence of medical abortion (i.e. non-surgical abortion using medications) as a safe and effective option has resulted in the further simplification of the appropriate standards and health worker skills required for safe abortion provision, making it possible to consider expanding the roles of a much wider range of health workers in the provision of safe abortion.

While shortages of all skilled health-care professionals exist, the deficits and subnational imbalances are the greatest for physicians. The 2013 World Health Organization (WHO) report on the global health workforce highlights the fact that advanced practitioners, midwives, nurses and auxiliaries are still insufficiently used in many settings. Involving such health workers makes it more likely that services will be available to women when they need them.

While WHO's 2012 publication *Safe abortion: technical and policy guidance for health systems* highlighted that abortion care can be safely provided by properly trained health-care providers, including non-physician providers who are trained in basic clinical procedures related to reproductive health, it did not provide specific recommendations with respect to different types of health workers or the tasks for which task shifting and task sharing are appropriate. There are no other global guidelines that provide such guidance, though some recommendations related to task shifting in contraceptive provision have been included in the *OptimizeMNH* recommendations, published in 2012. This guideline therefore aims to fill this gap with evidence-based recommendations on the safety, effectiveness, feasibility and acceptability of involving a range of health workers in the delivery of recommended and effective interventions for providing safe abortion and post-abortion care, including post-abortion contraception.

The guideline will be useful for policy-makers, implementers of national and subnational programmes, nongovernmental organizations and professional societies involved in the planning and management of such care. While policy and regulatory environments for safe abortion care may vary, abortion is legal at least to save the life of the woman in almost all countries, more than two thirds of countries have one or more additional grounds for legal abortion, and the provision of care for complications is always legal. Thus, the possibility of improving access to safe abortion or post-abortion care, or both, by expanding health worker roles exists in most contexts. The range of safe and effective options recommended here can facilitate evidence-based decision-making and adaptation to the context of local health workforce dynamics, resources and public health needs.

Process of guideline development

The guideline was developed according to the principles set out in the *WHO handbook for guideline development* and under the oversight of the Guidelines Review Committee of WHO. The core team at WHO (the Steering Group) was complemented by a team of experts on evidence synthesis from the Norwegian Knowledge Centre, Oslo, and by a multidisciplinary group of external technical experts who constituted the Guideline Development Group (GDG).

The tasks and health worker categories were defined based on insights from regional technical consultations and input from experts. Questions were developed in the population, intervention, comparator, outcome (PICO) format and priority outcomes (safety, effectiveness, satisfaction, acceptability and feasibility) were defined. A systematic search was conducted, review of the evidence was undertaken, and 36 studies that looked at effectiveness and 204 qualitative studies were included in the evidence base. Data came from both high-resource as well as low-resource settings. The certainty of the evidence on safety, effectiveness and satisfaction was assessed using the Grading of Recommendations Assessment, Development and Evaluation (GRADE) approach. Confidence in the qualitative findings on acceptability and feasibility were assessed using the Confidence in the Evidence from Reviews of Qualitative Research (CERQual) approach.

Recommendations were finalized in consultation with the GDG and using explicit Evidence to Decision (EtD) frameworks that considered benefits, harms, feasibility and acceptability, as well as resource use from the perspectives of women, the health system and health workers. Declarations of interest (DOIs) were managed according to standard procedures; no conflicts of interest were identified.

External peer reviewers, unconnected to the guideline development process, reviewed and critically appraised the draft guideline prior to its finalization.

Overview of recommendations

Recommendations have been made for tasks related to safe abortion care (including post-abortion contraception) and the management of complications of abortion (also known as post-abortion care in some settings and provided as part of emergency obstetric care). Only clinical interventions that have been recommended as safe and effective according to current WHO technical guidance (i.e. *Safe abortion: technical and policy guidance for health systems*) are included. The tasks are outlined in Table 1.

The range of types of health workers considered for the various tasks was broad-based and included specialist doctors (obstetrics and gynaecology), doctors not specialized in obstetrics and gynaecology, associate clinicians, midwives, nurses, auxiliary nurses (ANs) and auxiliary nurse midwives (ANMs), doctors of complementary systems of medicine (a significant portion of the workforce in some regions), pharmacists, pharmacy workers and lay health workers. Explanation of the categorization with illustrative examples can be found in Table 2.

Executive summary

One of the following types of recommendations has been made for each task and health worker combination:

Recommendation category	Symbol	Explanation
Recommended	✓	The benefits of implementing this option outweigh the possible harms. This option can be implemented, including at scale.
Recommended in specific circumstances	✓	The benefits of implementing this option outweigh the possible harms in specific circumstances. The specific circumstances are outlined for each recommendation. This option can be implemented under these specific circumstances.
Recommended in the context of rigorous research	R✓	There are important uncertainties about this option (related to benefits, harms, acceptability and feasibility) and appropriate, well designed and rigorous research is needed to address these uncertainties.
Recommended against	✗	This option should not be implemented.

All of the recommendations assume that the assigned health workers will receive task-specific training prior to implementation. The implementation of these recommendations also requires functioning mechanisms for monitoring, supervision and referral.

The recommendations are applicable in both high- and low-resource settings. They provide a range of options of types of health workers who can perform the specific task safely and effectively. The options are intended to be inclusive and do not imply either a preference for or an exclusion of any particular type of provider. The choice of a specific health worker for a specific task will depend upon the needs and conditions of the local context.

Health worker roles in providing safe abortion care and post-abortion contraception

Management of abortion and post-abortion care in the first trimester

	Lay health workers	Pharmacy workers	Pharmacists	Doctors of complementary systems of medicine	Auxiliary nurses/ANMs	Nurses	Midwives	Associate/advanced associate clinicians	Non-specialist doctors	Specialist doctors
Vacuum aspiration for induced abortion	✗**	✗**	✗**	✓	✓ (outside)	✓	✓	✓	✓*	✓*
Vacuum aspiration for management of uncomplicated incomplete abortion/miscarriage	✗**	✗**	✗**	✓ (outside)	✓ (outside)	✓	✓	✓	✓*	✓*
Medical abortion in the first trimester	Recommendation for subtasks (see below)	✗	Recommendation for subtasks (see below)	✓ (outside)	✓	✓	✓	✓	✓*	✓*
Management of uncomplicated incomplete abortion/miscarriage with misoprostol	R (recommendation)	✗	✗	✓ (outside)	✓	✓	✓	✓	✓*	✓*

* considered within typical scope of practice; evidence not assessed.
** considered outside of typical scope of practice; evidence not assessed.

Subtasks for medical abortion in the first trimester: No recommendation is made on the independent provision of medical abortion in the first trimester for pharmacists or lay health workers, but recommendations are made for subtasks as follows:

Subtasks for medical abortion in the first trimester

	Lay health workers	Pharmacists
Assessing eligibility for medical abortion	R✓	R✓
Administering the medications and managing the process and common side-effects independently	R✓	R✓
Assessing completion of the procedure and the need for further clinic-based follow-up	R✓	R✓

Health worker roles in providing safe abortion care and post-abortion contraception

Management of abortion and post-abortion care beyond 12 weeks

	Lay health workers	Pharmacy workers	Pharmacists	Doctors of complementary systems of medicine	Auxiliary nurses/ANMs	Nurses	Midwives	Associate/advanced associate clinicians	Non-specialist doctors	Specialist doctors
Dilatation and evacuation	✗**	✗**	✗**	✗	✗**	✗**	✗**	R	✓	✓*
Cervical priming (osmotic dilators)	✗**	✗**	✗**	✗	✗	✓	✓	✓	✓	✓*
Cervical priming (medications)	✗**	✗**	✗**	✓	✓	✓	✓	✓	✓*	✓*
Medical abortion > 12 weeks	✗**	✗**	✗**	✗	✗	✓	✓	✓	✓*	✓*

Management of non-life-threatening complications

	Lay health workers	Pharmacy workers	Pharmacists	Doctors of complementary systems of medicine	Auxiliary nurses/ANMs	Nurses	Midwives	Associate/advanced associate clinicians	Non-specialist doctors	Specialist doctors
Initial management of post-abortion infection	✗**	✗**	✗**	✓	✓	✓	✓	✓	✓*	✓*
Initial management of post-abortion haemorrhage	✗**	✗**	✗**	✓	✓	✓	✓	✓	✓*	✓*

* considered within typical scope of practice; evidence not assessed.
** considered outside of typical scope of practice; evidence not assessed.

Executive summary

Provision of post-abortion contraception

	Lay health workers	Pharmacy workers	Pharmacists	Doctors of complementary systems of medicine	Auxiliary nurses/ANMs	Nurses	Midwives	Associate/advanced associate clinicians	Non-specialist doctors	Specialist doctors
Insertion/removal of intrauterine devices (IUDs)	✗	✗	✗	✓ (SC)	✓ (for ANMs) / R (for auxiliary nurses)	✓	✓	✓*	✓*	✓*
Insertion/removal of implants	R	✗	✗	✓ (SC)	✓ (SC)	✓	✓	✓*	✓*	✓*
Initiation/continuation of injectable contraceptives	✓ (SC)	✓ (SC)	✓	✓	✓	✓	✓*	✓*	✓*	✓*
Tubal ligation	✗**	✗**	✗**	✗	✗	R	R	✓*	✓*	✓*

✓ = Recommended; ✓ (SC) = Recommended in specific circumstances; R = Recommend only in the context of rigorous research; ✗ = Not recommended

* considered within typical scope of practice; evidence not assessed.
** considered outside of typical scope of practice; evidence not assessed.

Health worker roles in providing safe abortion care and post-abortion contraception

Pre- and post-abortion counselling

	Lay health workers	Pharmacy workers	Pharma-cists	Doctors of comple-mentary systems of medicine	Auxiliary nurses/ ANMs	Nurses	Midwives	Associate/ advanced associate clinicians	Non-specialist doctors	Specialist doctors
Pre- and post-abortion counselling	✓	✗	✗	✓	✓	✓	✓	✓	✓*	✓*

Provision of information on safe abortion

	Lay health workers	Pharmacy workers	Pharma-cists	Doctors of comple-mentary systems of medicine	Auxiliary nurses/ ANMs	Nurses	Midwives	Associate/ advanced associate clinicians	Non-specialist doctors	Specialist doctors
Information on safe providers/ laws	✓	✓	✓	✓*	✓*	✓*	✓*	✓*	✓*	✓*

* considered within typical scope of practice; evidence not assessed.

Women themselves have a role to play in managing their own health and this constitutes another important component of task sharing within health systems. Therefore, the following recommendations were made related to self-assessment and self-management approaches in contexts where the woman has access to appropriate information and to health services should she need or want them at any stage of the process.

Role of self-management approaches

	Self
Medical abortion in the first trimester	No recommendation for overall task – recommendations for specific components as below
Self-assessing eligibility	R ✓
Managing the mifepristone and misoprostol medication without direct supervision of a health-care provider	✓
Self-assessing completeness of the abortion process	✓
Self-administering injectable contraception	✓

Research needs

The safety, effectiveness and feasibility of task sharing by health workers located outside of health-care facilities (i.e. in communities) or in pharmacies are important research areas for the future. Also critical is implementation research to identify effective strategies to implement task shifting at scale in national and subnational programmes.

Update and review

The recommendations in this guideline will be reviewed and updated in 2018.

Tasks and health workers considered in the guideline

Only tasks that have already been recommended as safe and effective in *Safe abortion: technical and policy guidance for health systems (3)* have been included.

The main task has been split into subtasks in some instances where it is clinically feasible for the subtasks to be performed as discrete and independent activities by different health workers, possibly at different locations or different time points.

Self-management and self-assessment approaches are included for some of the tasks as women themselves have an important role to play in the management of their own care. Such approaches can be empowering for women and also represent a way of optimizing available health workforce resources and sharing of tasks.

Table 1. Tasks and subtasks considered in the guideline

Specific tasks included in the scope of the guideline

Management of abortion and post-abortion care in the first trimester
• Vacuum aspiration for induced abortion
• Vacuum aspiration for the management of incomplete abortion
• Medical abortion with mifepristone + misoprostol or misoprostol alone, including the subtasks of:
  – assessment of eligibility
  – administration of medications and management of the process
  – assessment of abortion completeness
• Medical management of incomplete abortion with misoprostol
• Self-management of components of medical abortion

Management of abortion and post-abortion care beyond 12 weeks
• Dilatation and evacuation (D&E) for induced abortion, including specific subtasks as follows:
  – cervical priming with osmotic dilators
  – cervical priming with medications
• Medical abortion with mifepristone + misoprostol or misoprostol alone

Recognizing and managing non-life-threatening complications • Initial management of non-life-threatening post-abortion infection • Initial management of non-life-threatening post-abortion haemorrhage
Counselling and information provision • Provision of general information on safe providers, laws, contraception options • Pre- and post-abortion counselling
Post-abortion contraception provision • Insertion and removal of IUDs • Insertion and removal of implants • Initiation and continuation of injectable contraceptives • Tubal ligation (female sterilization)

The health worker types considered in the guideline are described in Table 2. The descriptions draw on a variety of sources including definitions used in the *OptimizeMNH* task-shifting guideline *(6)* and other WHO publications *(7–12)*.

Descriptions have been adapted to be generic enough to apply across settings. They are indicative and illustrative and are not intended to substitute formal definitions of professional bodies or those used in specific countries and are not official WHO definitions.

Table 2. Health worker category descriptions

Broad category	Illustrative description for the purpose of the tasks covered in this guideline	Examples
Specialist doctor	For the purpose of this guideline, specialization refers to postgraduate clinical training and specialization in obstetrics and gynaecology.	Gynaecologist, obstetrician
Non-specialist doctor	For the purpose of this guideline, this refers to a medical doctor who holds a university-level degree in basic medical education with or without further training in general practice or family medicine, but not in obstetrics and gynaecology.	Family doctor, general practitioner, medical doctor
Advanced associate and associate clinician	For the purpose of this guideline, this refers to a professional clinician with basic competencies to diagnose and manage common medical and surgical conditions and also to perform some types of surgery. Training can vary by country, but generally requires 3–4 years post-secondary education in an established higher education institution. The clinician is registered and his or her practice is regulated by a national or subnational regulatory authority.	Assistant medical officer, clinical officer, medical licentiate practitioner, health officer, physician assistant, surgical technician, non-physician clinician, medical assistant, nurse practitioner
Midwife	For the purpose of this guideline, this refers to a person who has been registered by a state midwifery or similar regulatory authority and has been trained in the essential competencies for midwifery practice. Training typically lasts 3 or more years in nursing or midwifery school and leads to a university degree or the equivalent. A registered midwife has the full range of midwifery skills.	Registered midwife, midwife, community midwife, nurse-midwife
Nurse	For the purpose of this guideline, this refers to a person who has been legally authorized (registered) to practice after examination by a state board of nurse examiners or similar regulatory authority. Education includes 3 or more years in nursing school, and leads to a university or postgraduate university degree or the equivalent.	Registered nurse, clinical nurse specialist, licensed nurse, BSc nurse
Auxiliary nurse midwife and auxiliary nurse	For the purpose of this guideline, an auxiliary nurse is someone trained in basic nursing skills but not in nursing decision-making. An auxiliary nurse midwife has basic nursing skills and some midwifery competencies but is not fully qualified as a midwife. The level of training may vary from a few months to 2–3 years. A period of on-the-job training may be included, and sometimes formalized in apprenticeships.	Auxiliary midwife, auxiliary nurse, ANMs, family welfare visitor

Table 2 (continued)

Broad category	Illustrative description for the purpose of the tasks covered in this guideline	Examples
Doctor of complementary systems of medicine	For the purpose of this guideline, this refers to a professional of traditional and complementary systems of medicine (non-allopathic physician) whose training includes a 4- or 5-year university degree that teaches the study of human anatomy, physiology, management of normal labour and the pharmacology of modern medicines used in obstetrics and gynaecology, in addition to their systems of medicine. For the purpose of this guideline, these doctors are included with reference to the provision of elements of abortion-related care as per conventional medical practice.	Ayush doctor, Ayurvedic physician, non-allopathic physician
Pharmacist	For the purpose of this guideline, this refers to a health practitioner who dispenses medicinal products. A pharmacist can counsel on the proper use and adverse effects of drugs and medicines following prescriptions issued by medical doctors/health professionals. Education includes university-level training in theoretical and practical pharmacy, pharmaceutical chemistry or a related field.	Pharmacist (USA), chemist (United Kingdom and the Commonwealth), clinical pharmacist, community pharmacist
Pharmacy worker	For the purpose of this guideline, this refers to technicians and assistants who perform a variety of tasks associated with dispensing medicinal products under the guidance of a pharmacist. They inventory, prepare and store medications and other pharmaceutical compounds and supplies, and may dispense medicines and drugs to clients and instruct on their use as prescribed by health professionals. Technicians typically receive 2–3 years training in a pharmaceutical school, with an award not equivalent to a university degree. Assistants have usually been through 2–3 years of secondary school with a subsequent period of on-the-job training or apprenticeship.	Pharmacy assistant, pharmacy technician dispenser, pharmacist aide, dispensary assistant
Lay health worker	For the purpose of this guideline, this refers to a person who performs functions related to health-care delivery/information provision and was trained in some way in the context of the task, but has received no formal professional or paraprofessional certificate or tertiary education degree.	Community health worker, village health worker, female community health volunteer

Background

Shortage of health-care professionals

Effective, safe and simple interventions for safe abortion and post-abortion care exist

Other relevant global guidelines

Objectives of this guideline

Background

Although simple, safe and effective interventions exist, 21.6 million unsafe abortions occur globally every year. Unsafe abortion continues to constitute a major mortality and morbidity burden especially in the developing world *(1)*. Numerous barriers limit access to safe abortion – one of the most critical is the lack of trained providers.

Shortage of health-care professionals

It is estimated that the global deficit of skilled health-care professionals (midwives, nurses and physicians) will be 12.9 million by 2035. As shown in Figure 1, 31 countries in Africa have a critically low (< 22.8/10 000 population) density of skilled health workers to population, but South-East Asia overall has the largest shortfall in absolute numbers because of the large populations in countries with critically low densities of health workers *(2)*. Not surprisingly, these are also the regions of the world with a particularly high burden of mortality related to unsafe abortion *(1)*.

Although deficits exist among all skilled health-care professionals, the shortages are more acute for physicians, and the population-based density of nurses and midwives is higher than that of physicians in most countries for which disaggregated data are available *(2)*.

Most countries, including many high-income countries, have additional subnational geographical imbalances in the availability of a skilled health workforce with a bias towards urban areas and/or the private sector. These disparities can result in inequities in access to health care.

Over and above the general shortages in the health workforce, in many settings the availability of trained providers may be further affected by the low priority given to preventing unsafe abortion, or by regulatory, policy and programmatic barriers to training, or the availability of supplies and commodities, or by the unwillingness of some health workers to provide abortion or post-abortion care (for a more complete discussion of barriers, refer to the document *Safe abortion: technical and policy guidance for health systems [3]*). Lack of trained providers disproportionately affects some women, leaving those who live in rural areas or are poor, less educated, young and unmarried particularly at risk of an unsafe abortion.

Health workers as defined by the World Health Organization (WHO) are:

> All people engaged in actions whose primary intent is to enhance health. This includes physicians, nurses and midwives, but also laboratory technicians, public health professionals, community health workers, pharmacists, and all other support workers whose main function relates to delivering preventive, promotive or curative health services.

This is a broad-based and inclusive definition, and as the report on the health workforce highlights, many types of health workers such as advanced practitioners, midwives, nurses and auxiliaries are still insufficiently used in many settings *(2, 4)*.

Effective, safe and simple interventions exist for safe abortion and post-abortion care

Task shifting and task sharing are plausible and feasible options as many of the interventions for safe abortion care, particularly those in early pregnancy, can be provided at the primary care level and on an outpatient basis *(3)*. While even vacuum aspiration is a primary care procedure, medical abortion (using pills) is non-invasive and simplifies the requirements of place, equipment and health worker skills. It is suggested that the WHO definition of unsafe abortion (an abortion performed by a person lacking the necessary skills or in an environment not in conformity with medical standards, or both) be reinterpreted in light of current technical evidence and to account for the differences in what constitutes a safe environment for these two methods *(5)*.

Health worker roles in providing safe abortion care and post-abortion contraception

Figure 1: Health workforce to population ratios in 186 countries

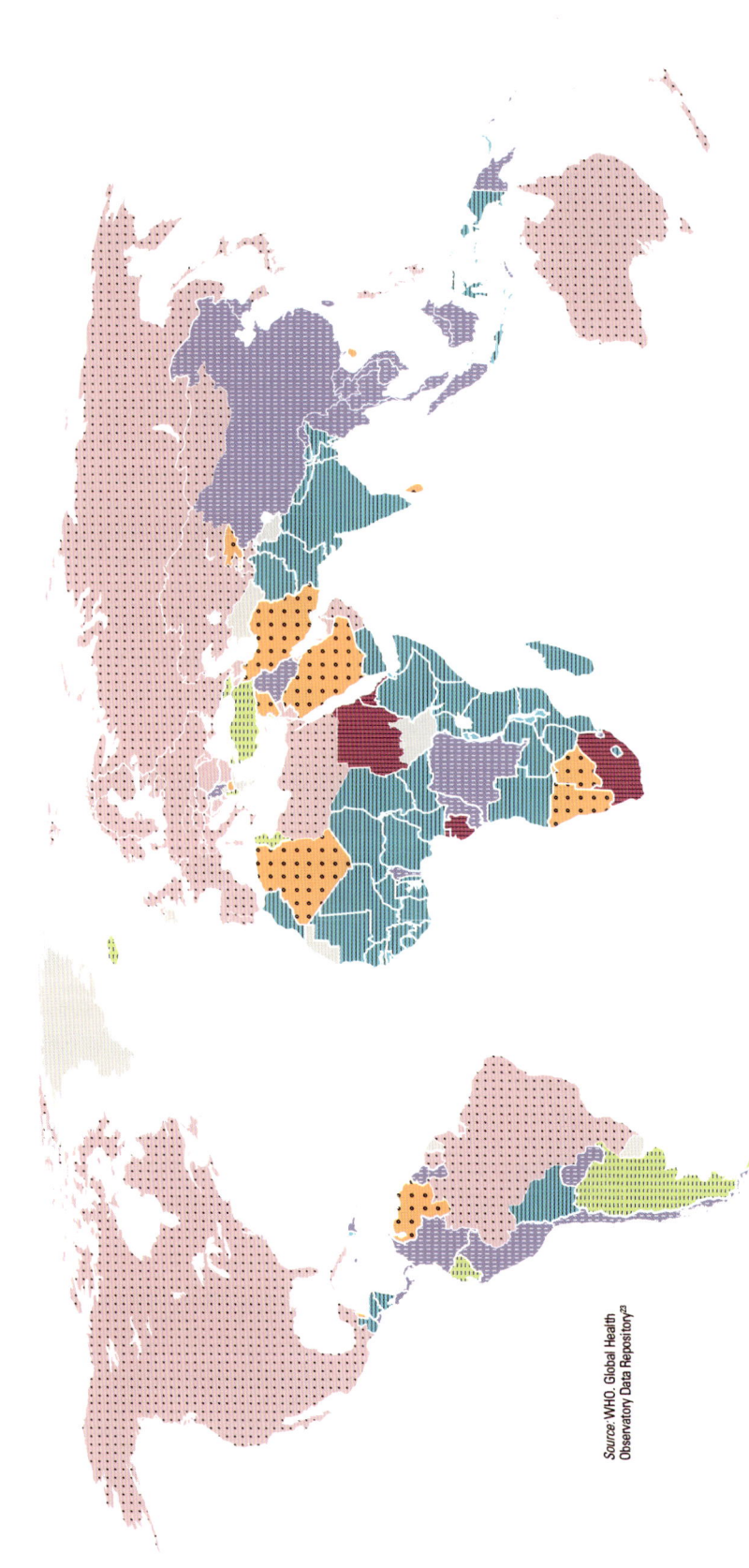

Group 1: density of skilled workforce lower than 22.8/10 000 population and a coverage of births attended by SBA less than 80%

Group 2: density of skilled workforce lower than 22.8/10 000 population and coverage of births attended by SBA greater than 80%

Group 3: density of skilled workforce lower than 22.8/10 000 population but no recent data on coverage of births attended by SBA

Group 4: density is equal or greater than 22.8/10 000 and smaller than 34.5/10 000

Group 5: density is equal or greater than 34.5/10 000 and smaller than 59.4/10 000

Group 6: density is equal or greater than 59.4/10 000

Source: WHO, 2013 (2); using data from Global Health Observatory Data Repository (online database), available at: http://apps.who.int/gho/data/

Other relevant global guidelines

The document *Safe abortion: technical and policy guidance for health systems (3; p. 65)* highlights the role of non-physician providers in the provision of safe abortion care, but it does not contain specific recommendations about the types of health workers and the tasks for which task shifting is appropriate.

The *OptimizeMNH* guideline *(6)* provides recommendations on task shifting for maternal and newborn health, but does not cover abortion and post-abortion care. It does, however, contain relevant recommendations for the provision of contraception by non-specialist providers. Where relevant, these have been incorporated into this guideline as well.

The need for specific recommendations on task shifting and task sharing in abortion care has been articulated by some WHO Member States and by stakeholders and experts in the field during the process of the dissemination of the safe abortion guidance document referred to above *(3)* and also during various technical consultations at WHO's Department of Reproductive Health and Research.

Objectives of this guideline

The primary objective of this guideline is to provide evidence-based recommendations on the safety, effectiveness, feasibility and acceptability of a range of health workers in the delivery of recommended and effective interventions for providing safe abortion and post-abortion care and in providing post-abortion contraception. These recommendations can be adapted to the context of local health workforce resources and the public health needs in the country of implementation.

The guideline is expected to be useful for:

- national and subnational policy-makers;
- implementers and managers of national and subnational reproductive health programmes;
- nongovernmental and other organizations and professional bodies involved in the planning and management of services for abortion and post-abortion care.

While legal, policy and regulatory contexts vary, abortion is legal at least to save the life of the woman in almost all countries and more than two thirds of countries have one or more additional grounds for legal abortion. The provision of care for complications (post-abortion care) is always legal. Thus, these recommendations are relevant across a diverse range of settings. They are also relevant in both high- and low-resource settings, as the need to make care more accessible and rationalize the use of available health resources exists in both these contexts.

How the guideline was developed

Contributors and their roles

Scoping and formulation of the guideline questions

Evidence retrieval and synthesis

Assessment of confidence in the evidence

Moving from evidence to recommendations

How the guideline was developed

The guideline was developed by the Department of Reproductive Health and Research at WHO in accordance with the *WHO handbook for guideline development (13)* and under the overall guidance of the WHO Guideline Review Committee.

Individuals from other organizations who contributed to this guideline did so in their capacity as individual experts. Donors to the Department who fund work on abortion issues were not included in the Guideline Development Group (GDG) and were not present at any of the GDG meetings. Commercial entities were not involved in developing the guideline nor was funding from such sources used.

Contributors and their roles

The work was coordinated by the Responsible Officer at the Department of Reproductive Health and Research. Within WHO, work on preventing unsafe abortion is housed solely within this Department, hence the WHO Steering Group comprised members of this Department, with additional representation from the Department of Maternal, Newborn, Child and Adolescent Health and from WHO regional offices. Inputs were sought from other units at WHO as needed. The Steering Group managed the day-to-day activities of developing the guideline, developed the guideline questions, participated in the evidence retrieval and synthesis, and developed the Evidence to Decision (EtD) frameworks and draft recommendations. The Responsible Officer drafted the guideline with input from the Core Evidence Team and Steering Group.

The Core Evidence Team comprised experts from the Norwegian Knowledge Centre, Oslo. They provided oversight on methodological issues and the evidence retrieval and syntheses, and were responsible for the GRADE and CERQual assessments of the certainty of evidence. They also worked with the Steering Group to draft the PICO questions and the EtD frameworks. Other experts provided technical input as needed. For example, an economist advised on resource use issues and an additional GRADE methodologist provided a second independent assessment of certainty.

The GDG comprised 18 members (10 women, 8 men) and included diverse expertise but with a particular focus on health systems and on regions of the world where the need for task sharing in abortion care is a high priority. The GDG provided input into the development of the scope of the guideline and the formulation of the questions and in reviewing the evidence and making recommendations. They also reviewed and approved the final guideline. In addition to ongoing consultations via email, Skype and GoToMeeting, two in-person meetings with the GDG were held in Geneva (November 2013 and October 2014).

Twelve individuals, external to the guideline development process and chosen to reflect end-users from priority regions or those with methodological expertise, served as external peer reviewers for the draft guideline.

Declarations of interest

All members of the GDG, the Core Evidence Team, peer reviewers and consultants were required to complete the standard WHO Declaration of Interest (DOI) form. GDG members completed the form prior to each of the meetings they attended and were also instructed to let the Secretariat know of any changes to their declared interests over time. The Steering Group evaluated the responses and discussed them with the Director of the Department. At the GDG meetings, the Chair presented a summary of the DOIs and all participants had the opportunity to confirm, append or amend any interests already declared.

Only two individuals – members of the GDG – declared secondary interests, which were not deemed to constitute a conflict of interest for the purpose of this guideline. No conflicts of financial interest or involvement with commercial entities were declared. The DOI forms have been electronically archived for future reference.

A complete list of all contributors, their affiliations, roles and DOIs is included in Annex A.

Scoping and formulation of the guideline questions

The initial list of tasks and health worker types to be considered for the guideline was developed on the basis of input and insights gained from previous technical consultations and regional meetings on safe abortion in Riga, Latvia (May 2012), Addis Ababa, Ethiopia (September 2012), Kathmandu, Nepal (September 2012), and Nairobi, Kenya (November 2012). Additionally, an online questionnaire was sent to a purposively selected group of approximately 90 knowledgeable individuals to help define some of the relevant health worker categories, country-level practices and health worker roles. Responses were received from 35 people many of whom provided further input on national policies relating to health worker roles. The preliminary list was finalized in consultation with the GDG.

Formulation of questions

Agreed on questions on health worker–task combinations were formulated in PICO (population, intervention, comparator, outcome) format. The prioritized outcomes were as follows:

- Benefits and harms:
  - safety: serious adverse events, complications (specific to the task);
  - effectiveness (specific to the task);
  - satisfaction of women receiving care with the overall services/health worker providing the care.
- Acceptability:
  - findings reported in qualitative research regarding the extent to which a task-shifting intervention is considered to be reasonable or adequate among women potentially or actually receiving abortion care, and among health workers potentially or actually delivering this care.
- Feasibility:
  - findings from qualitative studies on factors affecting implementation of task-shifting programmes at scale.

The specific operationalization of these concepts for each health worker–task combination can be found in the supplementary annexes (Web Supplement 2, Web Supplement 3).

Evidence retrieval and synthesis

Evidence for safety, effectiveness and satisfaction was drawn from randomized controlled trials, non-randomized controlled trials, controlled before-and-after studies and interrupted-time-series studies. Evidence for acceptability came from qualitative or mixed-method studies with a qualitative component. For the evidence on feasibility, all documented information related to task shifting in abortion care in five countries (Bangladesh, Ethiopia, Nepal, South Africa and Uruguay) was collected. The countries were selected to represent a diversity of regions and examples where national or subnational programmes on task shifting related to abortion care are already being implemented.

Existing reviews that directly or indirectly addressed the questions of interest were identified and their usefulness for this guideline was assessed before a search for further evidence was initiated. Seven reviews addressing effectiveness, two reviews addressing acceptability and a feasibility case study synthesis were undertaken specifically for this guideline. In addition, findings from three existing systematic reviews on effectiveness of pharmacists in providing other types of health interventions, and six existing qualitative systematic reviews and multicountry studies of the implementation of similar health worker programmes for other maternal health tasks were also incorporated into the evidence base.

Search strategies were specific to each question – they are described in full in the respective reviews in the web supplements (Web Supplement 2, Web Supplement 3). In general, databases were searched from inception to 2014, without language filters and for low- and middle-income as well as high-income countries. The databases searched included the following: African Index Medicus, Chinese Biomedical Literature Database, CINAHL, Cochrane Database, ClinicalTrials.gov, EBSCO, Embase, Global Index Medicus, Index Medicus for South-East Asia, Index Medicus for WHO Eastern Mediterranean Region, LILACS, Ovid MEDLINE, Popline, PubMed, Western Pacific Regional Index Medicus.

A special effort was made to identify and include non-English language literature for the acceptability/feasibility outcomes and most of the documented materials for the case study on Uruguay were in Spanish. Reference lists of key articles were also hand searched and external experts were contacted to identify additional relevant studies, including reports of completed trials that had not yet been published. For the case study synthesis, documented literature was supplemented with interviews with knowledgeable in-country experts.

Figure 2 charts the geographical spread of the data included in the evidence base.

Titles and abstracts were screened by two members of the review team and the full texts of shortlisted articles were further screened to determine if they met inclusion criteria.

For the safety and effectiveness findings, the GRADE profiler, GRADEpro,[1] was used to create evidence profiles and Summary of Findings tables. Forest plots were made to graphically illustrate the relative risk estimates. Meta-analyses were performed when more than one trial reported risk estimates relevant to outcomes. For qualitative reviews, two individuals identified the key findings relevant to the scope of the guidance. Findings were organized into Summary of Findings tables.

Figure 2: Informing the recommendations: the evidence base

Safety, effectiveness, satisfaction	Qualitative data on acceptability	Qualitative data on feasibility
36 studies from 18 countries • Africa – 4 • Eastern Mediterranean – 3 • Europe – 12 • Latin America – 2 • North America – 7 • South-East Asia – 13 • Western Pacific – 0	**83 studies from 24 countries** • Africa – 15 • Eastern Mediterranean – 0 • Europe – 10 • Latin America – 32 • North America – 12 • South-East Asia – 16 • Western Pacific – 2	**121 papers from 5 selected countries + in-depth interviews with in-country experts** • Bangladesh • Ethiopia • Nepal • South Africa • Uruguay

---

1 Available at: http://www.guidelinedevelopment.org/

Assessment of confidence in the evidence

The certainty (i.e. the extent to which one can be confident that an estimate of the effect or association is correct) of the benefits and harms outcomes was assessed using the GRADE approach. Five criteria – study limitations, consistency of effect, imprecision, indirectness and publication bias – were used to assess the certainty for each outcome. Evidence was downgraded by one level for serious and by two levels for very serious limitations. Assessments were made independently by two GRADE methodologists.

Confidence in findings from the reviews of qualitative studies was assessed with the CERQual tool, utilizing an approach similar to GRADE. Each review finding was assessed on four factors:

- the methodological limitations of the individual qualitative studies contributing to the review finding, assessed using an appropriate qualitative critical appraisal tool;
- the relevance of a review finding, assessed by the extent to which the supporting evidence is applicable to the context specified in the review question;
- the coherence of each review finding, assessed by the extent to which the review finding was based on data that were similar across multiple individual studies and/or incorporated convincing explanations for any variations;
- the adequacy of data supporting the review finding, assessed by determining the degree of richness and/or scope, as well as the quantity of data supporting a review finding.

An overall judgment of the confidence in each review finding was made, based on all of the above. Where existing systematic reviews were used, confidence assessments as reported in the original reviews were used. Assessing the confidence in each finding was not possible for the case study synthesis given that these findings were based on a wide range of evidence types.

Moving from evidence to recommendations

In order to follow a systematic process that explicitly considers the various factors that inform decisions on recommendations, the Evidence to Decision (EtD) frameworks developed by the DECIDE collaboration were used.[2]

One framework was prepared for each question using a pre-set template. All systematically synthesized evidence as well as additional information was summarized into the following sections:

- Background information:
  - This section contains information about the PICO, the context and general information about the task.
- Benefits and harms:
  - The section contains the Summary of Findings (SoF) tables on safety, effectiveness and satisfaction, a narrative description of the included studies, and relevant additional contextual information.
- Acceptability:
  - This section contains the summary of key findings from qualitative studies regarding the extent to which a task-shifting intervention is considered to be reasonable among women potentially or actually receiving abortion care and among health workers potentially or actually delivering this care. Acceptability to women was prioritized in decision-making; health worker acceptability informed implementation considerations.

---

2 DECIDE: http://www.decide-collaboration.eu/etd-evidence-decision-framework

- Feasibility:
  - This section contains the summary of key findings from qualitative research and from country case studies regarding the extent to which a task-shifting intervention is capable of being accomplished or implemented. The focus was on the feasibility of the intervention from a health system perspective, as well as on broader social, legal and political factors.
- Resources:
  - This section contains a summary of all resource-related outcomes reported within the studies that were selected for the safety and effectiveness evidence, and a qualitative assessment of resource needs in terms of training, supplies, referrals, supervision and monitoring, time and health worker remuneration. A health systems perspective was used in considering resource use, but especially for self-assessment and self-management approaches, resource use by women was also considered.
  - No formal cost analysis was conducted as such analyses tend to be very context specific; nor was a systematic search and evaluation of resource use information undertaken.
- Overall recommendations and decisions.
- Implementation considerations.
- Research needs.

Using the framework, separate judgments were made for each of the criteria; i.e. the balance of benefits and harms, acceptability, feasibility and resource use. The overall recommendation considered all of these factors as relevant. This is particularly important as this guideline is related to health systems.

The complete EtD frameworks are available in Web Supplement 1.

Use of the frameworks for decision-making

Draft EtD frameworks were prepared by the Steering Group and Core Evidence Team. These were reviewed by the GDG and recommendations finalized during the meeting in October 2014. In addition to the frameworks, the GDG also had access to all the evidence profiles and supplementary materials.

Decisions at the GDG meeting were consensus driven. The Chair allowed for discussion of differing views on recommendation options and the final decision was based on majority opinion, provided the panel members with opposing views were willing to agree to this outcome. An option for noting dissenting opinions was available, but it did not need to be used, nor did voting need to be resorted to.

Document preparation and peer review

The Responsible Officer at WHO worked with a consultant to write the draft guideline. The GDG reviewed the draft and their feedback was incorporated. The guideline was also reviewed by external peer reviewers unconnected with the process of guideline development. They provided structured feedback on accuracy, presentation, implementation considerations and on the overall usefulness of the guideline. No serious factual errors affecting recommendations were noted by the peer reviewers.

Recommendations

General considerations

Recommendation categories

Management of abortion and post-abortion care for pregnancies in the first trimester

Management of abortion and post-abortion care for pregnancies beyond 12 weeks

Management of non-life-threatening complications

Information about safe abortion and contraception

Pre- and post-abortion counselling

Provision of post-abortion contraception

Recommendations

General considerations

- The recommendations include tasks related to safe abortion care (including post-abortion contraception) and the management of complications of abortion (also known as post-abortion care in some settings and provided as part of emergency obstetric care).

- Recommendations about who can provide care have been made only for clinical interventions that have been recommended as safe and effective according to current WHO technical guidance i.e. *Safe abortion: technical and policy guidance for health systems (3).* The recommendations in this guideline should be implemented in accordance with the technical standards and human rights principles as laid down in that document.

- The recommendations are not targeted specifically to low-resource or low-income settings; they are intended for all settings where abortion-related care is provided.

- The recommendations are intended to be implemented within the context of functioning mechanisms for referral, monitoring and supervision, as well as access to the necessary equipment and commodities.

- The recommendations provide a range of options of types of health workers who can perform the specific task safely and effectively. The options are intended to be inclusive and do not imply either a preference for or an exclusion of any particular type of provider. The specific choice of health workers depends upon the needs and conditions of the local context.

It is also important to note that the following assumption underlies all the options that have been recommended in this guideline:

- It is assumed that any health worker discussed in this guideline has the basic training required of that type of health worker. In addition, the recommendations all assume that health workers will receive the training or information specific to the task, prior to implementation of the recommendation option.

It is important to interpret all of the recommendations that follow in the context of these general considerations and assumptions.

Recommendation categories

Four types of recommendations are made:

Recommended

✅ The benefits of implementing this option outweigh the possible harms. This option can be implemented including at scale.

For certain health worker–task combinations, the GDG decided that the option was within the typical scope of practice of the health worker. No assessment of evidence was made in such cases and this has been noted in the justification.

Recommended in specific circumstances

 The benefits of implementing this option outweigh the possible harms in specific circumstances. The specific circumstances are outlined for each recommendation. This option can be implemented under these specific circumstances.

Recommended in the context of rigorous research

Ⓡ There are important uncertainties about this option (related to benefits, harms, acceptability and feasibility) and appropriate, well designed and rigorous research is needed to address these uncertainties.

Recommended against

❌ This form of task shifting should not be implemented.

For certain health worker–task combinations, the GDG decided that the option was outside the typical scope of practice of the health worker. No assessment of evidence was made in such cases and this has been noted in the justification.

The explanation and justification for each recommendation is provided and the certainty of the evidence has been indicated where appropriate as follows:

- **High certainty**: Further research is very unlikely to change our confidence in the estimate of effect.
- **Moderate certainty**: Further research is likely to have an important impact on our confidence in the estimate of effect and may change the estimate.
- **Low certainty**: Further research is very likely to have an important impact on our confidence in the estimate of effect and is likely to change the estimate.
- **Very low certainty**: We are very uncertain about the estimate.

Confidence assessments of qualitative research evidence are referred to in the following terms:

- **High confidence**: It is highly likely that the review finding is a reasonable representation of the phenomenon of interest.
- **Moderate confidence**: It is likely that the review finding is a reasonable representation of the phenomenon of interest.
- **Low confidence**: It is possible that the review finding is a reasonable representation of the phenomenon of interest.
- **Very low confidence**: It is not clear whether the review finding is a reasonable representation of the phenomenon of interest.

Management of abortion and post-abortion care for pregnancies in the first trimester

Manual or electric vacuum aspiration, as well as medical abortion with mifepristone followed by misoprostol (or misoprostol alone in contexts where mifepristone is not available), are appropriate methods to terminate a pregnancy in the first trimester. Uncomplicated incomplete abortion (both induced and spontaneous) can be managed with manual vacuum aspiration (MVA) or electric vacuum aspiration (EVA), or with oral or sublingual misoprostol.

Vacuum aspiration for induced abortion

The provision of vacuum aspiration includes the assessment of gestational age, cervical priming (if needed), the actual procedure, pain management including the provision of a paracervical block (if needed) and the assessment of completeness of abortion through the visual inspection of products. Health workers with the skills to perform a bimanual pelvic examination to diagnose and date a pregnancy, and to perform a transcervical procedure such as intrauterine device (IUD) insertion, can be trained to perform vacuum aspiration *(3)*. The recommendations are presented in Table 3.

Table 3. Recommendations for vacuum aspiration for induced abortion*

Health worker	Recommendation	Justification
Specialist doctors, non-specialist doctors	Recommended	Within their typical scope of practice. No assessment of the evidence was therefore conducted.
Associate and advanced associate clinicians	Recommended	There is evidence for the safety and effectiveness (moderate certainty) and for women's satisfaction with the overall abortion experience (low certainty). This option is feasible in both high- and low-resource settings, and may decrease inequities by extending safe abortion care to underserved populations.
Midwives	Recommended	There is evidence for the safety and effectiveness (moderate certainty) and for women's satisfaction with the overall abortion experience (low certainty). This task is recognized as a core competency in midwifery. Women often consider care received from midwives as more supportive (moderate confidence). The option has been shown to be feasible, including in low-resource settings.
Nurses	Recommended	There is evidence for the safety and effectiveness (low certainty) and for women's satisfaction with this option (low certainty). Women often consider care received from nurses as more supportive (moderate confidence). The option is feasible and may decrease inequities by extending safe abortion care to underserved populations.

Table 3 (continued)

Health worker	Recommendation	Justification
Auxiliary nurses (AN) and auxiliary nurse midwives (ANM)	Recommended in specific circumstances ✓ We recommend this option in contexts where established mechanisms to include ANMs/ANs in providing basic emergency obstetric care or post-abortion care already exist.	Although there was insufficient direct research evidence for the effectiveness of this option, the benefits outweigh any possible harms. The option has also been shown to be feasible, including at scale in low-resource settings, and has the potential to decrease inequities by extending safe abortion care to rural and underserved populations.
Doctors of complementary systems of medicine	Recommended in specific circumstances ✓ We recommend this option in contexts with established health system mechanisms for the participation of doctors of complementary systems of medicine in other tasks related to maternal and reproductive health.	There is evidence for the effectiveness of components of the task, e.g. assessing uterine size with bimanual examination as part of medical abortion provision (low certainty). These professionals perform transcervical procedures such as IUD insertion in some settings. The benefits outweigh possible harms and the option has the potential to increase equitable access to safe abortion care in regions where these professionals constitute a significant proportion of the health workforce.
Pharmacists, pharmacy workers, lay health workers	Recommended against ✗	Outside of their typical scope of practice. No assessment of the evidence was therefore conducted.

* Refer to MVA1 and EVA1 framework in Web Supplement 1 (p. 5) for summary of evidence.

Additional remarks

While MVA is more commonly used and more likely in primary care settings, the skills required for EVA are similar, thus the recommendations above apply to the provision of either form of vacuum aspiration.

There may be more procedural difficulties in pregnancies of over nine weeks duration. In experienced hands the procedure can be used in pregnancies up to 14 weeks; however, for all health worker types, more training and experience is needed for the use of MVA at 12–14 weeks pregnancy duration as compared to the use of MVA at < 12 weeks.

Implementation considerations

The vacuum aspiration procedure can be performed in a primary care facility and on an outpatient basis.

Recommendations

Management of uncomplicated incomplete abortion using vacuum aspiration

Managing uncomplicated incomplete abortion with MVA/EVA (when uterine size is less than 13 weeks) includes recognizing the condition, assessing uterine size, the actual procedure and pain management. Table 4 gives the recommendations.

Table 4. Management of uncomplicated incomplete abortion/miscarriage in the first trimester with vacuum aspiration*

Health worker	Recommendation	Justification
Specialist doctors, non-specialist doctors	Recommended ✓	Within their typical scope of practice. No assessment of the evidence was therefore conducted.
Associate and advanced associate clinicians	Recommended ✓	There is evidence for the safety and effectiveness of the provision of vacuum aspiration for induced abortion (moderate certainty; see Table 3) by these health workers. The skills required for the management of uncomplicated incomplete abortion with vacuum aspiration are similar.
Midwives	Recommended ✓	There is evidence for the safety and effectiveness of the provision of vacuum aspiration for induced abortion (moderate certainty; see Table 3) by these health workers. The skills required for the management of uncomplicated incomplete abortion with vacuum aspiration are similar. The option appears to be feasible, including in low-resource settings.
Nurses	Recommended ✓	There is evidence for the safety and effectiveness of the provision of vacuum aspiration for induced abortion (low certainty; see Table 3) by these health workers. The skills required for the management of uncomplicated incomplete abortion with vacuum aspiration are similar. The option appears to be feasible, including in low-resource settings.
Auxiliary nurses and auxiliary nurse midwives	Recommended in specific circumstances ✓ We recommend this option in contexts where established health systems mechanisms involve ANMs/ANs in providing basic emergency obstetric care, and where referral and monitoring systems are strong.	There was insufficient direct research evidence for the safety and effectiveness of this option. However, the option of this type of health worker delivering emergency obstetric care (which includes removing retained products as a signal function) or post-abortion care using MVA has been shown to be feasible in programmes in several low-resource settings.

Table 4 (continued)

Health worker	Recommendation	Justification
Doctors of complementary systems of medicine	Recommended in specific circumstances ✓ We recommend this option in contexts with established health system mechanisms for the participation of doctors of complementary systems of medicine in other tasks related to maternal and reproductive health.	There is evidence for the effectiveness of carrying out components of the task, e.g. assessing uterine size with bimanual examination as part of medical abortion provision (low certainty). These professionals perform transcervical procedures like IUD insertion in some settings. This option has the potential to increase equitable access to safe abortion care in regions where these professionals constitute a significant proportion of the health workforce.
Pharmacists, pharmacy workers, lay health workers	Recommended against ✗	Outside of their typical scope of practice. No assessment of the evidence was therefore conducted.

* Refer to MVA2 and EVA2 framework in Web Supplement 1 (p. 17) for summary of evidence.

Additional remarks

While MVA is more commonly used and more likely in primary care settings, the skills required for EVA are similar; thus the recommendations above apply to the provision of either form of vacuum aspiration.

Uncomplicated incomplete abortion can result after an induced or spontaneous abortion (i.e. miscarriage). The management is identical and the above recommendations apply to both situations.

Implementation considerations

The evacuation of retained products is also a signal function of basic emergency obstetric care and training and implementation can be integrated with emergency obstetric care (EmOC) services.

Medical abortion in the first trimester

Medical abortion (MA) refers to the sequential use of mifepristone followed by misoprostol or, in settings where mifepristone is not available, the use of misoprostol alone. The specific dosage, routes and regimens are different at differing pregnancy durations and are detailed in the *Clinical practice handbook for safe abortion (14)*.

MA is a process that takes place over a period of several days rather than being a discrete procedure. The process includes several components or subtasks:

- assessing eligibility for MA (diagnosing and dating the pregnancy, ruling out medical contraindications, screening for possible ectopic pregnancy);
- administering the medications with instructions on their appropriate use and managing the common side-effects;
- assessing that the abortion process is complete and that no further intervention is required.

One health worker can provide the entire package, but it is equally possible for the subtasks to be performed by different health workers and at different locations. See Table 5 for the recommendations.

Table 5. The provision of medical abortion (MA) in the first trimester*

Health worker	Recommendation	Justification
Specialist doctors, non-specialist doctors	Recommended ✓	Within their typical scope of practice. No assessment of the evidence was therefore conducted.
Associate and advanced associate clinicians	Recommended ✓	There is evidence for the effectiveness of carrying out components of the task, e.g. assessing gestation as part of MVA provision. There is also evidence that health worker types with similar or less comprehensive basic training (e.g. midwives, nurses, auxiliary nurse midwives) can provide MA safely and effectively (moderate certainty). The option is feasible and the potential to expand access to underserved populations is high.
Midwives	Recommended ✓	There is evidence for the safety and effectiveness of this option (moderate certainty). More women are satisfied with the provider when midwives provide MA (moderate certainty). The option appears feasible and is already being implemented in several countries.
Nurses	Recommended ✓	There is evidence for the safety and effectiveness, and for women's satisfaction with abortion services with this option (moderate certainty).
Auxiliary nurses and auxiliary nurse midwives	Recommended ✓	There is evidence for the safety and effectiveness (moderate certainty) of this option. The option appears feasible and is already being implemented in some low-resource settings.

Table 5 (continued)

Health worker	Recommendation	Justification
Doctors of complementary systems of medicine	Recommended in specific circumstances ✓ We recommend this option only in contexts with established health system mechanisms for the participation of doctors of complementary systems of medicine in other tasks related to maternal and reproductive health.	There is evidence for the safety and effectiveness, and for women's satisfaction with this type of provider and services (low certainty). The benefits outweigh any possible harms, and the potential to reduce inequities in access to safe abortion care in regions where such professionals form a significant proportion of the health workforce is high.
Pharmacists	No recommendation for independent provision of MA; see Table 6 for recommendations made for subtasks.	Before making a recommendation on full independent provision of MA it is necessary to demonstrate the effectiveness and feasibility of the subtasks.
Pharmacy workers	Recommended against ✗	There was no evidence for the safety, effectiveness, acceptability or feasibility of this option. However, it is important to note that as with all other drugs and medications, pharmacy workers should dispense mifepristone and misoprostol as indicated by prescription.
Lay health workers	No recommendation for the overall package; see Table 7 for recommendations made for subtasks.	Before making a recommendation on full independent provision of MA it is necessary to demonstrate the safety and feasibility of carrying out the subtasks.

* Refer to MA1 and subtasks framework in Web Supplement 1 (p. 25) for summary of evidence.

Additional remarks
Available evidence for the independent provision of MA by non-physicians is for pregnancy durations up to 10 weeks (70 days). Further research is needed on pregnancies of 11–12 weeks.

It is not essential that the person providing the MA should also be trained and competent in MVA provision. However, in such cases, backup referral access to a provider who can perform MVA if needed should be ensured. Such backup does not necessarily have to be at the same site.

Implementation considerations
Restrictions on prescribing authority for some categories of providers may need to be modified or other mechanisms put in place for allowing such providers to administer the MA medications within the regulatory framework of the health system.

There is a higher chance of ongoing pregnancy when misoprostol alone is used; hence, irrespective of the level of provider, training has to emphasize the ability to detect these cases for further management/referral.

Subtasks for medical abortion

No recommendations are made regarding the independent provision of MA in the first trimester for pharmacists or lay health workers, but recommendations were made for specific subtasks of MA provision, as presented in Tables 6 and 7.

Table 6. The provision of medical abortion subtasks in the first trimester by pharmacists*

Subtask	Recommendation	Justification
Assessing eligibility for medical abortion	Recommended within the context of rigorous research	The approach has the potential to improve the triage of health care by screening and referral to appropriate health-care facilities. Rigorous research on this approach using simple tools and checklists is needed to address the uncertainties and to test the feasibility of the option in a programme setting.
Administering the medications and managing the process and common side-effects independently	Recommended within the context of rigorous research	Dispensing medications on prescription is within the typical scope of practice of these health workers and should be continued. However, well designed research is still needed on the effectiveness and feasibility in a programme setting of the approach of pharmacists independently making clinical judgments related to managing the process and its common side-effects. The approach has the potential to improve access as pharmacies are often women's first point of contact with the health system; however, the feasibility of developing referral linkages with the health system also needs to be studied.
Assessing completeness of the procedure and the need for further clinic-based follow-up	Recommended within the context of rigorous research	This option has the potential to improve the triage of health care by screening women in need of further care. Research on this approach using simple tools like urine pregnancy tests and checklists is needed, as is research to test the feasibility of the option in a programme setting.

* Refer to MA1 and subtasks – Pharmacists and pharmacy workers framework in Web Supplement 1 (p. 35) for summary of evidence.

Table 7. The provision of medical abortion subtasks in the first trimester by lay health workers*

Subtask	Recommendation	Justification
Assessing eligibility for medical abortion	Recommended within the context of rigorous research	Fewer women may be assessed as eligible when lay health workers assess eligibility for medical abortion using simple checklists (low certainty). However, the option is promising and lay health workers are often involved, either formally or informally, in advising women who are seeking such care (moderate confidence). Well designed research is needed to refine the optimum tools and checklists needed and to test the feasibility in community settings.
Administering the medications and managing the process and common side-effects.	Recommended within the context of rigorous research	The option has the potential to expand access to safe care, and well designed research has the potential to address any uncertainties around safety, effectiveness and feasibility.
Assessing completeness of the procedure and the need for further clinic-based follow-up	Recommended within the context of rigorous research	There is evidence that lay health workers can accurately assess abortion completeness using simple checklists (low certainty). Approaches using a urine pregnancy test as part of the assessment toolkit could yield better results and require further research.

* Refer to MA1 and subtasks – Lay health workers framework in Web Supplement 1 (p. 43) for summary of evidence.

Additional remarks

Strong referral linkage and backup care to emergency services must always be available as part of the research. Initial research should focus on pregnancy durations of 10 weeks (70 days) or less.

As with all other drugs and medications, dispensing mifepristone and misoprostol on prescription is within the typical scope of practice of pharmacists and the research recommendation above is not intended to imply any change in that scope of practice.

Recommendations

Self-management of the medical abortion process in the first trimester

Given the nature of the medical abortion (MA) process, it is possible for women to play a role in managing some of the components by themselves outside of a health-care facility. Such self-assessment and self-management approaches can be empowering for women and help to triage care, leading to a more optimal use of health resources. See the recommendations in Table 8.

Table 8. Women's role in managing the process of medical abortion*

Woman's role	Recommendation	Justification
Managing the entire process of medical abortion up to 84 days	No recommendation for the overall package; recommendations made for subtasks as below.	Individual components of the self-management of medical abortion have been tested; however, there is as yet insufficient evidence on using all three components together.
Self-assessing eligibility for medical abortion	Recommended within the context of rigorous research ®	Women may be more conservative in assessing eligibility using simple checklists (low certainty). However, the approach is promising and further work is needed on developing appropriate assessment tools.
Managing the mifepristone and misoprostol medication without direct supervision of a health-care provider	Recommended in specific circumstances ✓ We recommend this option in circumstances where women have a source of accurate information and access to a health-care provider should they need or want it at any stage of the process.	There is evidence that the option is safe and effective (low-certainty evidence from numerous studies, but using non-randomized designs given the strong preferences of women for one or the other option). More women report the method to be satisfactory when it is self-managed (low certainty). Women find the option acceptable and feasible (high confidence) and providers also find the option feasible (high confidence).
Self-assessing completeness of the abortion process using pregnancy tests and checklists	Recommended in specific circumstances ✓ We recommend this option in circumstances where both mifepristone and misoprostol are being used and where women have a source of accurate information and access to a health-care provider should they need or want it at any stage of the process.	There is evidence that the option is safe and effective including in low-literacy, low-resource settings (moderate to high certainty).

* Refer to MA3 and subtasks in Web Supplement 1 (p. 51) for summary of evidence.

Additional remarks

A follow-up visit after MA using mifepristone–misoprostol is not mandatory *(3)*. The efficacy of MA is lower when misoprostol alone is used; hence the self-assessment of completeness when misoprostol alone is used requires further research.

Available evidence for managing the medications and process without direct supervision of the provider is for pregnancy durations of nine weeks (63 days) or less.

Self-management approaches reflect an active extension of health systems and health care. These recommendations are NOT an endorsement of clandestine self-use by women without access to information or a trained health-care provider/health-care facility as a backup. All women should have access to health services should they want or need it.

Implementation considerations

Mechanisms to ensure access and linkages to post-abortion contraception services need to be established.

Management of uncomplicated incomplete abortion with misoprostol

Managing uncomplicated incomplete abortion with misoprostol (when uterine size is up to 13 weeks) includes recognizing the condition, assessing uterine size and administering oral or buccal misoprostol in the correct dose. Table 9 gives the recommendations on this.

Table 9. Management of uncomplicated incomplete abortion/miscarriage in the first trimester with misoprostol*

Health worker	Recommendation	Justification
Specialist doctors, non-specialist doctors	Recommended ✓	Within their typical scope of practice. No assessment of the evidence was therefore conducted.
Associate and advanced associate clinicians	Recommended ✓	There is moderate-certainty evidence for the safety and effectiveness of medical management of incomplete abortion by midwives and moderate-certainty evidence for the effectiveness of medical abortion provision by health worker types with similar or less comprehensive basic training. Additionally, there is direct evidence that these health workers can assess gestational age as part of MVA provision. The option is feasible and the potential to expand access to underserved populations is high.
Midwives	Recommended ✓	There is evidence from a low-resource setting for the safety and effectiveness (moderate certainty) of this option and for women's overall satisfaction with the provider (moderate certainty) when midwives manage incomplete abortion. The option appears feasible and has the potential to reduce inequities in access to safe abortion.
Nurses	Recommended ✓	There is evidence for the safety, effectiveness and satisfaction of providing medical abortion (moderate certainty; see Table 5), and the skills required for managing incomplete abortion with misoprostol are similar. The option appears feasible and has the potential to reduce inequities in access to safe abortion.
Auxiliary nurses and auxiliary nurse midwives	Recommended ✓	There is evidence for the safety and effectiveness of the provision of medical abortion in the first trimester (moderate certainty; see Table 5), and the skills required for managing incomplete abortion with misoprostol are similar.

Table 9 (continued)

Health worker	Recommendation	Justification
Doctors of complementary systems of medicine	Recommended in specific circumstances ✓ We recommend this option only in contexts with established health system mechanisms for the participation of doctors of complementary systems of medicine in other tasks related to maternal and reproductive health.	There is evidence for the safety and effectiveness of the provision of medical abortion in the first trimester (low certainty; see Table 5), and the skills required for managing incomplete abortion with misoprostol are similar.
Pharmacists and pharmacy workers	Recommended against ✗	There was insufficient evidence for the safety and effectiveness of this option. It is also not within the typical scope of practice of pharmacists or pharmacy workers to conduct a full evaluation to diagnose incomplete abortion or determine uterine size.
Lay health workers	Recommended within the context of rigorous research (R)	There was no direct evidence for this option, but there is some evidence that lay health workers can use simple tools and checklists to determine gestational age or abortion completeness (low certainty). Such health workers are often involved in advising women seeking such care (moderate confidence). In general, lay health worker interventions are acceptable and have proved feasible in many contexts. The further development of tools and carrying out rigorous research can help to address some of the uncertainties associated with this option.

* Refer to MA2 framework in Web Supplement 1 (p. 60), MA2 – Pharmacists and pharmacy workers framework in Web Supplement 1 (p. 68) and MA2 – Lay health workers framework in Web Supplement 1 (p. 74) for summaries of evidence.

Additional remarks
Uncomplicated incomplete abortion can result after an induced or spontaneous abortion (i.e. miscarriage). The management is identical and the above recommendations apply to both situations.

Implementation considerations
Restrictions on prescribing authority for some categories of providers may need to be modified or other mechanisms put in place for making the medications available for these providers within the regulatory framework of the health system.

The evacuation of retained products is a signal function of basic EmOC; thus training and implementation of these tasks can be integrated with EmOC services.

Research needs
Research into lay health worker roles in carrying out this task requires the documentation of safety and effectiveness of their ability to recognize uncomplicated incomplete abortions, to administer the correct dose of misoprostol and to recognize and refer if other complications are present. Strong referral linkage and backup care to emergency services must always be available.

Management of abortion and post-abortion care for pregnancies beyond 12 weeks

Dilatation and evacuation (D&E) and medical abortion with mifepristone followed by misoprostol (or misoprostol alone in contexts where mifepristone is not available) are the recommended options *(3, 14)*. The recommendations are given in Table 10.

Dilatation and evacuation (D&E)

Table 10. Provision of D&E for pregnancies beyond 12 weeks*

Health worker	Recommendation	Justification
Specialist doctors	Recommended ✓	Within their typical scope of practice. No assessment of the evidence was therefore conducted.
Non-specialist doctors	Recommended ✓	There was no direct evidence for the safety or effectiveness of this option as compared to specialist doctors. However, it appears to be feasible in both high- and low-resource settings where D&E use is common. Such doctors also routinely perform other surgical procedures like caesarean section, vacuum extraction and tubal ligation. The potential benefits of this option outweigh the harms. A specialist provider may not always be available on-site and this option may increase the ability of the health system to provide care for women needing it.
Associate and advanced associate clinicians	Recommended within the context of rigorous research ®	There was no direct evidence for the safety or effectiveness. However, the potential benefits outweigh the possible harms and the option has the potential to reduce inequities in access and increase the likelihood of facilities being able to provide care in the second trimester. It is therefore important to test this option under research conditions.
Doctors of complementary systems of medicine	Recommended against ✗	There was no direct evidence for the safety, effectiveness or feasibility of this option. The procedure requires skills beyond what is required for vacuum aspiration in pregnancies up to 12 weeks and the procedure is usually performed at facilities where specialist or non-specialist doctors are available.
Midwives, nurses, nurse-midwives, auxiliary nurse midwives, pharmacists, pharmacy workers, lay health workers	Recommended against ✗	Outside of their typical scope of practice. No assessment of the evidence was therefore conducted.

* Refer to D&E framework in Web Supplement 1 (p. 80) for summary of evidence.

Additional remarks
Whatever the level of provider, skills needed for D&E provision are greater than for a MVA/EVA done in earlier pregnancy and training needs are significantly higher.

Implementation considerations
Although usually performed at a higher-level facility, the procedure can still be done on an outpatient basis.

Health workers providing, or caring for women undergoing, abortion in the second trimester may have additional needs for professional and mentoring support.

Subtask: cervical priming

Cervical preparation with osmotic dilators or medications is recommended for all women undergoing D&E. Cervical priming is not mandatory at lower pregnancy duration but it can be used.

Osmotic dilators are placed 6–24 hours prior to the procedure. As such, placement can be performed by a health professional other than the provider who will conduct the D&E. If mifepristone is used it is given orally 24–48 hours before the procedure; if misoprostol is being used it is given sublingually or vaginally 2–3 hours before. Thus it is possible for priming to be initiated by a provider other than the one performing the D&E. The recommendations are given in Tables 11 and 12.

Table 11. Cervical priming with osmotic dilators prior to D&E*

Health worker	Recommendation	Justification
Specialist doctors, non-specialist doctors	Recommended	Within their typical scope of practice. No assessment of the evidence was therefore conducted.
Associate and advanced associate clinicians	Recommended in specific circumstances We recommend that this option be implemented if the priming is initiated under supervision of the health-care provider responsible for performing the D&E.	There is evidence for the safety and effectiveness of EVA/MVA provision (moderate certainty), which included cervical priming with osmotic dilators for select cases. This option may help optimize workflow within a facility and decrease waiting times for women.
Midwives	Recommended in specific circumstances We recommend that this option be implemented if the priming is initiated under supervision of the health-care provider responsible for performing the D&E.	Although there was insufficient direct evidence for this option, midwives are recommended to do other transcervical procedures like inserting an IUD, and there is evidence that provision of MVA by midwives is effective and safe (moderate certainty; see Table 3). This option may help optimize workflow within a facility and decrease waiting times for women.

Table 11 (continued)

Health worker	Recommendation	Justification
Nurses	Recommended in specific circumstances ✓ We recommend that this option be implemented if the priming is initiated under supervision of the health-care provider responsible for performing the D&E.	Although there was insufficient direct evidence for this option, nurses are recommended to do other transcervical procedures like inserting an IUD, and there is evidence that the provision of MVA by nurses is safe and effective (moderate certainty; see Table 3). This option may help optimize workflow within a facility and decrease waiting times for women.
Auxiliary nurses and auxiliary nurse midwives	Recommended against ✗	There was insufficient direct evidence for the safety and effectiveness of this option. These health workers are unlikely to be involved in second trimester abortion care.
Doctors of complementary systems of medicine	Recommended against ✗	There was insufficient direct evidence for the safety and effectiveness of this option. These health workers are unlikely to be involved in second trimester abortion care.
Pharmacists, pharmacy workers, lay health workers	Recommended against ✗	Outside of their typical scope of practice. No assessment of the evidence was therefore conducted.

*Refer to PRIME1 framework in Web Supplement 1 (p. 86) for summary of evidence.

Table 12. Cervical priming with medications prior to D&E*

Health worker	Recommendation	Justification
Specialist doctors, non-specialist doctors	Recommended ✓	Within their typical scope of practice. No assessment of the evidence was therefore conducted.
Associate and advanced associate clinicians	Recommended in specific circumstances ✓ We recommend this option be implemented if the priming is initiated under supervision of the health-care provider responsible for performing the D&E.	There is evidence for health workers with similar or less comprehensive basic training (e.g. midwives, nurses, ANMs) using such medications to provide medical abortion (moderate certainty), and cervical priming is part of the training for MVA provision.
Midwives	Recommended in specific circumstances ✓ We recommend this option be implemented if the priming is initiated under supervision of the health-care provider responsible for performing the D&E.	There is evidence for the safety and effectiveness of midwives being able to use these medications to provide medical abortion (moderate certainty, see Table 5), and cervical priming is part of the training for MVA provision.
Nurses	Recommended in specific circumstances ✓ We recommend this option be implemented if the priming is initiated under supervision of the health-care provider responsible for performing the D&E.	There is evidence for the safety and effectiveness of nurses providing medical abortion using these medications (moderate certainty; see Table 5), and cervical priming is part of the training for MVA provision.

Table 12 (continued)

Health worker	Recommendation	Justification
Auxiliary nurses and auxiliary nurse midwives	Recommended in specific circumstances ✓ We recommend this option be implemented if the priming is initiated under supervision of the health-care provider responsible for performing the D&E.	There is evidence for the safety and effectiveness of these health workers providing medical abortion using these medications (moderate certainty; see Table 5), and cervical priming is also part of the training for MVA provision.
Doctors of complementary systems of medicine	Recommended in specific circumstances ✓ We recommend this option be implemented if the priming is initiated under supervision of the health-care provider responsible for performing the D&E.	There is evidence for the safety and effectiveness of these health workers providing medical abortion using these medications (low certainty; see Table 5), and cervical priming is also part of the training for MVA provision.
Pharmacists, pharmacy workers	Recommended against ✗	Although dispensing medications with a prescription is within the scope of practice of pharmacists, this procedure is for use in facility-based second trimester abortion.
Lay health workers	Recommended against ✗	This procedure is for use in conjunction with a facility-based second trimester abortion. Lay health workers are unlikely to be involved with second trimester abortion care.

* Refer to PRIME2 framework in Web Supplement 1 (p. 93) and PRIME2 – Pharmacists and pharmacy workers framework in Web Supplement 1 (p. 99) for summaries of evidence.

Provision of medical abortion for pregnancies beyond 12 weeks

The provision of medical abortion for pregnancies beyond 12 weeks is a facility-based procedure and women should remain under observation until the process is complete. Table 13 presents the recommendations for health worker roles.

Table 13. Provision of medical abortion beyond 12 weeks*

Health worker	Recommendation	Justification
Specialist doctors	Recommended ✓	Within their typical scope of practice. No assessment of the evidence was therefore conducted.
Non-specialist doctors	Recommended ✓	There was insufficient direct evidence for this option; however, non-specialist doctors routinely carry out tasks of similar or greater complexity (e.g. conducting deliveries, manual removal of placenta, vacuum extraction). The potential benefits of this option outweigh the harms and the intervention has proven feasible in several settings. A specialist provider may not always be available on-site and this option may increase the ability of the health system to provide care for women needing it.
Associate and advanced associate clinicians	Recommended in specific circumstances ✓ We recommend this option in contexts where established and easy access to appropriate surgical backup and proper infrastructure is available to address incomplete abortion or other complications.	There was insufficient direct evidence for this option; however, such professionals are considered as options for tasks of similar complexity, like vacuum extraction and manual removal of placentas *(6)*. They are often present at higher-level facilities where second trimester care is provided. A trained specialist provider may not always be present at such a facility and the potential to sustain second trimester services is increased with more than one trained provider on site.
Midwives	Recommended in specific circumstances ✓ We recommend this option in contexts where established and easy access to appropriate surgical backup and proper infrastructure to address incomplete abortion or other complications is available.	Although there was insufficient direct evidence for the effectiveness of the intervention as a whole, midwives are often responsible for the monitoring and care of the woman from the time of misoprostol administration to completion of abortion, and women often find care provided by midwives to be more acceptable (moderate confidence).

Table 13 (continued)

Health worker	Recommendation	Justification
Nurses	Recommended in specific circumstances ✓ We recommend this option in contexts where established and easy access to appropriate surgical backup and proper infrastructure is available to address incomplete abortion or other complications.	Although there was insufficient direct evidence for the effectiveness of the intervention as a whole, nurses are often responsible for the monitoring and care of the woman from the time of misoprostol administration to completion of abortion, and women often find care provided by nurses to be more acceptable (moderate confidence).
Auxiliary nurses and auxiliary nurse midwives	Recommended against ✗	There was no direct evidence for the effectiveness, safety or acceptability of this option. These health workers are unlikely to be present at the higher-level facilities where such care is provided or be involved in second trimester abortion care.
Doctors of complementary systems of medicine	Recommended against ✗	There was no direct evidence for the effectiveness, safety or acceptability of this option. These doctors are unlikely to be involved in second trimester abortion care and the procedure is performed at a higher-level facility where specialist/non-specialist doctors are usually present.
Pharmacists, pharmacy workers, lay health workers	Recommended against ✗	Outside of their typical scope of practice. No assessment of the evidence was therefore conducted.

* Refer to MA4 framework in Web Supplement 1 (p. 104) for summary of evidence.

Research priorities
Further research is needed into the roles of non-physician providers – such as associate and advanced associate clinicians, midwives and nurses – for carrying out second trimester abortions.

Implementation considerations
Medical abortions for pregnancies beyond 12 weeks need to take place in health-care facilities with provision for inpatient stay.

Health workers providing, or caring for women undergoing, abortion in the second trimester may have additional needs for professional and mentoring support.

Management of non-life-threatening complications

Initial and basic management includes recognizing the complication, stabilizing the woman, providing oral or parenteral antibiotics and intravenous fluids prior to referral to an appropriate health-care provider/facility to provide definitive care (see Tables 14 and 15).

Table 14. Initial management of non-life-threatening post-abortion infection*

Health worker	Recommendation	Justification
Specialist doctors, non-specialist doctors	Recommended ✓	Within their typical scope of practice. No assessment of the evidence was therefore conducted.
Associate and advanced associate clinicians, midwives, nurses, auxiliary nurses and auxiliary nurse midwives	Recommended ✓	Although there was no direct evidence for the management of post-abortion infection, the management of puerperal sepsis with intramuscular (IM) antibiotics, which requires similar skills, is recommended as being within the typical scope of practice of these health workers *(6)*.
Doctors of complementary systems of medicine	Recommended in specific circumstances ✓ We recommend this option only in contexts with established health system mechanisms for the participation of doctors of complementary systems of medicine in other tasks related to maternal and reproductive health.	There was no direct evidence for the management of post-abortion infection, but the basic training of these professionals covers the skills required for this task.
Pharmacists, pharmacy workers, lay health workers	Recommended against ✗	Outside of their typical scope of practice. No assessment of the evidence was therefore conducted.

*Refer to COMP1 framework in Web Supplement 1 (p. 111) for summary of evidence.

Additional remarks
More specific recommendations relating to the comprehensive management of post-abortion infection were not made due to lack of clinical guidelines on the management of complications from unsafe abortion.

Implementation considerations
Restrictions on prescribing authority for some categories of providers may need to be modified or other mechanisms put in place for allowing such providers to administer the antibiotic medications within the regulatory framework of the health system.

Table 15. Initial management of non-life-threatening post-abortion haemorrhage*

Health worker	Recommendation	Justification
Specialist doctors, non-specialist doctors	Recommended ✓	Within their typical scope of practice. No assessment of the evidence was therefore conducted.
Associate and advanced associate clinicians, midwives, nurses	Recommended ✓	Although there was no direct evidence for the management of post-abortion haemorrhage, the initial management of post-partum haemorrhage with intravenous (IV) fluids, which requires similar skills, is considered as being within their typical scope of practice *(6)*.
Auxiliary nurses and auxiliary nurse midwives	Recommended ✓	Although there was no direct evidence for the management of post-abortion haemorrhage, the initial management of post-partum haemorrhage with IV fluids, which requires similar skills, is a recommended task *(6)*.
Doctors of complementary systems of medicine	Recommended in specific circumstances ✓ We recommend this option only in contexts with established health system mechanisms for the participation of doctors of complementary systems of medicine in other tasks related to maternal and reproductive health.	There was no direct evidence for the management of post-abortion haemorrhage, but the basic training of these professionals covers the skills required for this task.
Pharmacists, pharmacy workers, lay health workers	Recommended against ✗	Outside of their typical scope of practice. No assessment of the evidence was therefore conducted.

* Refer to COMP2 in Web Supplement 1 (p. 111) for summary of evidence.

Additional remarks
More specific recommendations for comprehensive management were not made due to lack of clinical guidelines on the management of complications from unsafe abortion.

Recommendations

Information about safe abortion and contraception

This section considers the provision of general information related to safe abortion care, for example: where and how to obtain methods of contraception; where and how to obtain safe, legal abortion services and cost information; specifics of local laws; and the importance of seeking care early. This information could be provided to women seeking these services but also to other women or men. The recommended options are given in Table 16.

Table 16. Provision of information on safe abortion*

Health worker	Recommendation	Justification
Specialist doctors, non-specialist doctors, associate and advanced associate clinicians, doctors of complementary systems of medicine, midwives, nurses, auxiliary nurses and auxiliary nurse midwives	Recommended ✓	Within their typical scope of practice. No assessment of the evidence was therefore conducted.
Pharmacists	Recommended ✓	There is evidence for the effectiveness of provision of education and counselling on chronic illnesses (low to moderate certainty). These professionals are often consulted by women seeking advice on how to deal with delayed menstruation (moderate confidence). Pharmacists are qualified professionals and routinely provide information about medications.
Pharmacy workers	Recommended in specific circumstances: ✓ We recommend this option only in contexts where it can be ensured that the pharmacy worker is under the direct supervision of a pharmacist and where access to a referral linkage with a formal health system exists	There was insufficient direct evidence for the effectiveness, safety and acceptability of this option. However, in many contexts, such workers are often consulted by women seeking information on how to deal with delayed menstruation (moderate confidence). Even though the effectiveness of training interventions with such workers is uncertain, the potential benefits of such workers being able to provide basic information outweighs the potential harms of them not providing information or providing incorrect information.
Lay health workers	Recommended ✓	Lay health worker interventions in health promotion are generally well accepted and feasible in many contexts where there is a strong lay health worker programme (moderate confidence). The potential to expand equitable access to information and safe abortion care is high.

* Refer to MESSAGE1 – Pharmacists and pharmacy workers framework in Web Supplement 1 (p. 119) and MESSAGE1 – Lay health workers in Web Supplement 1 (p. 127) for summaries of evidence.

Pre- and post-abortion counselling

The provision of scientifically accurate and easy-to-understand information to all women undergoing an abortion, and non-directive voluntary counselling to women who request it, is a core element of good quality abortion services. Comprehensive contraceptive information and services should be routinely integrated with abortion and post-abortion care *(15)*. However, counselling is more than information provision and refers to a focused, interactive process through which the woman voluntarily receives support, information and non-directive guidance from a trained person *(14)*. It requires a much higher level of specific knowledge than providing general information about safe abortion care. Table 17 gives the recommendations.

Table 17. Provision of pre- and post-abortion counselling*

Health worker	Recommendation	Justification
Specialist doctors, non-specialist doctors	Recommended ✓	Within their typical scope of practice. No assessment of the evidence was therefore conducted.
Associate and advanced associate clinicians	Recommended ✓	This task is a core element of provision of abortion or post-abortion care.
Midwives	Recommended ✓	Counselling is a core competency for midwives and this task is a core element of provision of abortion or post-abortion care.
Nurses, auxiliary nurses and auxiliary nurse midwives	Recommended ✓	This task is a core element of provision of abortion or post-abortion care.
Doctors of complementary systems of medicine	Recommended in specific circumstances ✓ We recommend this option only in contexts with established health system mechanisms for the participation of doctors of complementary systems of medicine in other tasks related to maternal and reproductive health.	This task is a core element of provision of abortion or post-abortion care.

Table 17 (continued)

Health worker	Recommendation	Justification
Pharmacists	Recommended against ❌	Although pharmacists are qualified to provide information about the drugs they dispense and there is evidence of effectiveness (low certainty) in counselling patients on the management of chronic conditions, their scope of practice does not include surgical options, thus they are not well placed to provide counselling on all safe abortion/contraception methods. Additionally, pharmacies may not be suitable places in terms of the privacy required for providing pre- and post-abortion counselling, hence this option may not be feasible in most settings.
Pharmacy workers	Recommended against ❌	There was no evidence for the safety, effectiveness or feasibility of this approach.
Lay health workers	Recommended in specific circumstances ✅ We recommend this option in limited circumstances in contexts where the health-care provider managing the procedure is unavailable to provide counselling or the woman needs additional support.	There was insufficient direct evidence for the effectiveness, acceptability and feasibility of this option, but lay health worker interventions are generally well accepted and feasible in many contexts, and lay health workers are often intermediaries between the formal health systems and women seeking abortion-related care (moderate confidence). These workers could play a supportive role to the main provider or counsellor.

* Refer to MESSAGE2 framework in Web Supplement 1 (p. 133), MESSAGE2 – Pharmacists and pharmacy workers in Web Supplement 1 (p. 119) and MESSAGE2 – Lay health workers in Web Supplement 1 (p. 127) for summaries of evidence.

Provision of post-abortion contraception

Contraception can be initiated immediately post-abortion and all contraceptive options may be used. Criteria laid out in the *Medical eligibility criteria for contraceptive use (16)* and principles of voluntary contraceptive provision within a human rights framework *(15)* should be adhered to.

See Tables 18 to 22 for the recommendations on the methods covered. Although a full consideration of all methods was outside the scope of this guideline, this does not imply that post-abortion contraceptive options for women should be limited to the methods listed below.

Intrauterine device

Table 18. Insertion and removal of an intrauterine device*

Health worker	Recommendation	Justification
Specialist doctors, non-specialist doctors, associate and advanced associate clinicians	Recommended ✓	The recommendation comes from the *OptimizeMNH* guideline *(6)* where this task was considered as being within the typical scope of practice of these health workers.
Midwives and nurses	Recommended ✓	The recommendation comes from the *OptimizeMNH* guideline *(6)*.
Auxiliary nurse midwives	Recommended ✓	The recommendation comes from the *OptimizeMNH* guideline *(6)*.
Auxiliary nurses	Recommended within the context of rigorous research ®✓	The recommendation comes from the *OptimizeMNH* guideline *(6)*.
Doctors of complementary systems of medicine	Recommended in specific circumstances ✓ We recommend this option only in contexts with established health system mechanisms for the participation of doctors of complementary systems of medicine in other tasks related to maternal and reproductive health.	Their basic training generally covers the relevant skills needed for this task. This option is probably feasible and may promote continuity of care for women and increase access in regions where such professionals form a significant proportion of the health workforce.
Pharmacists and pharmacy workers	Recommended against ✗	There was no direct evidence for the safety, effectiveness, acceptability or feasibility of this option.
Lay health workers	Recommended against ✗	The recommendation comes from the *OptimizeMNH* guideline *(6)*.

* Refer to CONTRA1 – Doctors of complementary systems of medicine framework in Web Supplement 1 (p. 138) and CONTRA1 – Pharmacists and pharmacy workers framework in Web Supplement 1 (p. 144) for summaries of evidence.

Recommendations

Implants

Table 19. Insertion and removal of implants*

Health worker	Recommendation	Justification
Specialist doctors, non-specialist doctors, associate/advanced associate clinicians	Recommended ✓	The recommendation comes from the *OptimizeMNH* guideline *(6)* where this task was considered as being within the typical scope of practice of these practitioners.
Midwives and nurses	Recommended ✓	The recommendation comes from the *OptimizeMNH* guideline *(6)*.
Auxiliary nurses and auxiliary nurse midwives	Recommended in specific circumstances ✓ We recommend this option within the context of targeted monitoring and evaluation.	The recommendation comes from the *OptimizeMNH* guideline *(6)*.
Doctors of complementary systems of medicine	Recommended in specific circumstances ✓ We recommend this option only in contexts with established health system mechanisms for the participation of doctors of complementary systems of medicine in other tasks related to maternal and reproductive health and where training in implant removal is given along with training in insertion.	There was insufficient direct evidence for the effectiveness of this option. However, the basic training of this cadre covers the relevant skills needed for this task. This option may promote continuity of care for women.
Pharmacists and pharmacy workers	Recommended against ✗	There was no direct evidence for the safety, effectiveness, acceptability or feasibility of this option.
Lay health workers	Recommended within the context of rigorous research (R)	The recommendation comes from the *OptimizeMNH* guideline *(6)*.

* Refer to CONTRA1 – Doctors of complementary systems of medicine framework in Web Supplement 1 (p. 138) and CONTRA1 – Pharmacists and pharmacy workers framework in Web Supplement 1 (p. 144) for summaries of evidence.

Additional remarks

The removal of implants can require greater skills than insertion and any health worker trained to independently insert implants should also be well trained on implant removal.

Research on the role of lay health workers in the insertion and removal of implants should be limited to lay health workers who deliver care within a health-care facility or other setting with sterile conditions *(6)*.

Injectable contraception

Table 20. Initiation and continuation of injectable contraceptives*

Health worker	Recommendation	Justification
Specialist doctors, non-specialist doctors, associate/advanced associate clinicians, midwives, nurses	Recommended ✓	The recommendation comes from the *OptimizeMNH* guideline *(6)* where this task was accepted as being within the typical scope of practice of these practitioners.
Auxiliary nurses and auxiliary nurse midwives	Recommended ✓	The recommendation comes from the *OptimizeMNH* guideline *(6)*.
Doctors of complementary systems of medicine	Recommended in specific circumstances ✓ We recommend this option only in contexts with established health system mechanisms for the participation of doctors of complementary systems of medicine in other tasks related to maternal and reproductive health.	The basic training of this cadre covers the relevant skills needed for this task, hence additional training needs would be minimal. This option may promote continuity of care for women.
Pharmacists	Recommended ✓	Although the available evidence for effectiveness is of very low certainty, administering injections is within the typical scope of practice of pharmacists and the additional training needs for this task would be minimal. This option has the potential to increase women's choices and reduce inequities in contraceptive access.

Table 20 (continued)

Health worker	Recommendation	Justification
Pharmacy workers	Recommended in specific circumstances ✓ We recommend this option only in contexts where the pharmacy worker is administering injectable contraceptives under direct supervision of a pharmacist.	There was no evidence for the effectiveness, acceptability or feasibility of this option. However, administering injections is within the typical scope of practice for trained pharmacy workers, thus the additional training needs would be not be high. This option has the potential to increase women's choices and reduce inequities in contraceptive access.
Lay health workers	Recommended in specific circumstances ✓ We recommend this option be implemented under targeted monitoring and evaluation.	The recommendation comes from the *OptimizeMNH* guideline *(6)*.

* Refer to CONTRA1 – Doctors of complementary systems of medicine Web Supplement 1 (p. 138) and CONTRA1 – Pharmacists and pharmacy workers framework in Web Supplement 1 (p. 144) for summaries of evidence.

Implementation considerations

Setting up adequate mechanisms for the disposal of used sharps, syringes and needles is important and particularly relevant when involving pharmacists and pharmacy workers as pharmacies may not have such mechanisms in place.

The investment in initial training may be higher where pharmacists are not already certified to provide injections. Mechanisms to link the pharmacist to the formal health system and ensure a referral linkage are important.

Research priorities

Since the research evidence for pharmacists is from high-resource settings, implementation research on feasibility issues in low-resource settings is needed.

Self-administration of injectable contraception

In addition, recommendations are made on the self-administration of injectable contraceptives by women themselves (see Table 21).

Table 21. Self-administration of injectable contraception*

Self-administration of injectable contraceptives	Recommendation	Justification
Women (self-administration)	Recommended in specific circumstances ✓ We recommend this option in contexts where mechanisms to provide the woman with appropriate information and training exist, referral linkages to a health-care provider are strong, and where monitoring and follow-up can be ensured.	There is evidence from high-resource settings that continuation rates for self-administered injectable contraceptives are similar to injectable contraceptives being provided by clinic-based providers (low certainty). The option may result in time and financial savings for women. There is evidence that some women prefer self-injection and the option may increase choice and autonomy in contraceptive use within a rights-based framework.

*Refer to CONTRA1 – Self-administration framework in Web Supplement 1 (p. 152) for summaries of evidence.

Additional remarks

The administration of an injectable contraceptive involves using a standard syringe and may be intramuscular or subcutaneous. Compact pre-filled auto-disable devices are still not widely available.

Implementation considerations

The following are important considerations when making the self-injection option available:

- adequate arrangements for storage and for keeping sharps safely at home;
- training in and the provision of mechanisms for the safe and secure disposal of used injectable contraceptives (especially in settings with high HIV prevalence);
- ensuring a way to procure injectable contraceptives on a regular basis without needing to repeatedly visit a health-care facility.

Recommendations

Tubal ligation

Table 22. Tubal ligation

Health worker	Recommendation	Justification
Specialist doctors, non-specialist doctors, associate/ advanced associate clinicians	Recommended ✅	The recommendation comes from the *OptimizeMNH* guideline *(6)* where this task was accepted as being within the typical scope of practice of these practitioners.
Midwives and nurses	Recommended within the context of rigorous research Ⓡ✓	The recommendation comes from the *OptimizeMNH* guideline *(6)*.
Auxiliary nurses and auxiliary nurse midwives	Recommended against ❌	The recommendation comes from the *OptimizeMNH* guideline *(6)*.
Doctors of complementary systems of medicine	Recommended against ❌	Outside of their typical scope of practice. No assessment of the evidence was therefore conducted.
Pharmacists, pharmacy workers	Recommended against ❌	Outside of their typical scope of practice. No assessment of the evidence was therefore conducted.
Lay health workers	Recommended against ❌	The recommendation comes from the *OptimizeMNH* guideline *(6)* where this task was accepted as being outside of the typical scope of practice of these practitioners.

Research needs and implementation considerations

Research needs

General implementation considerations

Research needs and implementation considerations

Research needs

A formal research prioritization exercise was not possible, but priority areas for future research were identified, including documenting the safety, effectiveness and feasibility of approaches to expanding roles of pharmacists and lay health workers in performing components of medical abortion provision. Further research is also needed into the development of simple tools, tests and checklists that can facilitate the assessment of eligibility for early medical abortion or of abortion completeness by women themselves or other community-based health workers.

Research is also needed into the safety, effectiveness and feasibility of non-specialist providers such as associate and advanced associate clinicians, midwives and nurses in providing abortion care beyond the first trimester.

Equally critical is implementation research on interventions to expand health worker roles within health systems and at scale, and to identify what works and what does not.

Given that task shifting and task sharing already exist in many contexts, more rigorous documentation and evaluation of existing programmes and the roles played by different types of health workers can also provide much-needed feasibility evidence. Programmes, as well as research (including clinical research), should clearly document and make visible the roles of health workers who provide the various interventions.

General implementation considerations

Implementation considerations specific to individual tasks have been highlighted along with the relevant recommendation in the preceding chapters.

A complete discussion of the implementation considerations for safe abortion care is given in *Safe abortion: technical and policy guidance for health systems (3)* and in the *Clinical practice handbook for safe abortion (14)*. Considerations for the implementation of contraceptive services can be found in *Ensuring human rights in the provision of contraceptive information and services (15)*. A discussion of general considerations for task shifting in maternal health and family planning can be found in the *OptimizeMNH guideline (6)*. Findings from the qualitative reviews on acceptability and feasibility undertaken for this guideline also identified numerous facilitators and barriers to implementation; a complete summary of these findings is presented in Web Supplement 3.

It is essential that task shifting and the overall expansion of health worker roles takes place as part of a planned and regulated strategy accompanied by appropriate mechanisms for training, certification and ongoing monitoring and support, and not as an opportunistic or de facto transfer of tasks because of the unavailability or the reluctance of a particular group of professionals to provide care.

Stakeholder involvement and working with professional associations across different levels of health worker groups is important in fostering trust, support for complementary roles and to create an enabling environment. The perceptions and attitudes of particular stakeholders can greatly influence the implementation of task shifting for abortion care. Addressing the concerns of more specialized providers who may be uncomfortable about shifting or sharing of tasks traditionally within their domain is important, as is addressing the concerns of health workers who will need to take on these additional roles. The latter may have legitimate concerns about workloads, remuneration and professional roles, and may also not always be supportive of or willing to be involved in providing abortion or post-abortion care or contraception.

Competency-based training is a key prerequisite in building confidence and preparing health workers for new roles. The learning curve required for a new skill to be fully acquired, and therefore the time lag needed for newly introduced interventions to reach optimum effectiveness, should not be underestimated. Over time, mechanisms to include the training in pre-service curricula are important to sustain task shifting at scale.

The training must address not only the specific tasks but also issues related to abortion and contraception more broadly, including an understanding of local laws. Training must aim to promote respectful care for women irrespective of the personal beliefs of individual health workers. Conscientious objection, where allowed, should be regulated, and provision of alternate care for the woman ensured.

Changes need to be developed in regulatory structures or mechanisms for health workers to access the necessary commodities and supplies within a health system setting.

Implicit in the implementation of these recommendations is the shift of services for early abortion care to the primary care level. Initial investments in strengthening the infrastructure to make that shift are likely to result in long-term gains. Self-management approaches and the involvement of pharmacists or lay health workers requires special attention to creating referral linkages (as these may not exist) and developing training materials and tools, and mechanisms for a supply of quality drugs within a regulated and monitored health systems context.

Ongoing supportive mentoring is needed as well. Health workers providing care related to abortion may face additional stigma or professional isolation in some contexts and mechanisms for support are therefore particularly important, especially for health workers involved with second trimester abortion care and those working in rural areas.

Ensuring retention of trained health workers in rural or underserved areas can be particularly challenging. This requires, among other things, giving professional and personal support, ensuring security for health workers and providing adequate remuneration and non-monetary rewards. The guideline on *Increasing access to health workers in remote and rural areas through improved retention (17)*, though not directly addressing the issue of abortion, contains relevant recommendations that may be useful when implementing the recommendations of this guideline.

Effective implementation requires a functioning health system. However, the need for being inclusive of a range of health-care providers can often be even more acute in contexts where health systems are dysfunctional or disrupted (e.g. in humanitarian or crisis settings) and task shifting for abortion and contraception-related care in such settings should not be overlooked.

Guideline dissemination, adaptation, monitoring and review

Dissemination and adaptation of the guideline

Monitoring guideline use

Review and update of the guideline

Guideline dissemination, adaptation, monitoring and review

Dissemination and adaptation of the guideline

The complete guideline along with all supplementary and additional information is available online[3] and in print, and can also be accessed through the WHO Library database, the WHO Sexual and Reproductive Health web page and the WHO Reproductive Health Library (RHL)[4].

The in-print English version of the guideline will be followed by Spanish and French versions. Translations into other UN languages will be developed as needed. Third-party translations into additional non-UN languages are encouraged, provided they comply with WHO guidance on such translations.

Additionally, a simplified summary of the recommendations is available in print and online and through an interactive web application.

Print copies will be distributed as per the standardized distribution lists maintained by WHO, and distribution and dissemination of additional copies will be coordinated with WHO regional offices and through active collaboration with donors, other agencies and partner nongovernmental organizations (NGOs). Regional dissemination workshops are planned, as is active dissemination at the FIGO World Congress and other international meetings. Implementation research activities are being prioritized, especially as related to the identified research needs.

Technical support for the adaptation and implementation of this guideline in countries will be provided at the request of ministries of health or WHO regional or country offices.

Monitoring guideline use

The number of print copies distributed as well as the number of downloads from the WHO website will be used as an indicator of interest in this guideline. Requests received for technical support for adaptation will be monitored, as will adoption of these recommendations in national guidelines and those of professional bodies and NGOs.

The GDG will work with the Secretariat to keep WHO informed of such events; an online survey will be conducted through WHO regional and country offices and with selected respondents of other user groups (e.g. professional societies, NGOs) two years after guideline publication in order to gauge in-country adoption and implementation of the recommendations. This survey will also help in gathering feedback relevant to future modifications.

Review and update of the guideline

The guideline will be reviewed in 2018 (four years after the evidence retrieval and synthesis was conducted for this guideline) unless new evidence warrants changes in existing recommendations earlier than this planned review date.

---

3 Available at: www.who.int/reproductivehealth/publications/unsafe_abortion/abortion-task-shifting/en/
4 The WHO Library database is available at: http://www.who.int/library/databases/en/; WHO's Sexual and Reproductive Health web page is available at: http://www.who.int/reproductivehealth/topics/unsafe_abortion/en/; WHO's RHL is available at: http://apps.who.int/rhl/en/